- Reach for a book instead of the remote . . . (Remember, books don't come with snack-food commercials!)

- Start a reading group . . . and serve a fresh-fruit salad.

- Try going to sleep earlier . . . it'll cut down on binges *and* make you more attractive, relaxed, and alert the next day.

- Give yourself a steamy, scented bath and a luxurious home facial . . . you'll feel so pretty you won't mind passing up the potato chips.

Find tips like these—and many more—in . . .

101 Ways to Stop Eating After Dinner

101
Ways to Stop Eating After Dinner

NANCY BUTCHER

BERKLEY BOOKS, NEW YORK

NOTICE: Every effort has been made to ensure that the information contained in this book is complete and accurate. However, neither the publisher nor the author is engaged in rendering professional advice or services to the individual reader. The ideas, procedures, and suggestions contained in this book are not intended as a substitute for consulting with your physician. All matters regarding your health require medical supervision. Neither the author nor the publisher shall be liable or responsible for any loss, injury or damage allegedly arising from any information or suggestion in this book.

101 WAYS TO STOP EATING AFTER DINNER

A Berkley Book / published by arrangement with the author

PRINTING HISTORY
Berkley edition / February 2001

The Penguin Putnam Inc. World Wide Web site address is http://www.penguinputnam.com

ISBN: 0-425-18095-6

BERKLEY®
Berkley Books are published by The Berkley Publishing Group, a division of Penguin Putnam Inc., 375 Hudson Street, New York, New York 10014.
BERKLEY and the "B" design are trademarks belonging to Penguin Putnam Inc.

PRINTED IN THE UNITED STATES OF AMERICA

10 9 8 7 6 5 4 3 2 1

Contents

Why You Need This Book

Just about every diet expert and diet program will tell you to stop eating after dinner or not to eat anything after 7:00 or 8:00 P.M.

Why? Because research suggests that the later you eat, the greater the chance your body will store that food as fat.

The problem is, these experts never tell you *how* to stop. And we all know how tough those hours before bedtime can be. They're a snacking temptation land mine, and the downfall of many dieters.

You know what I'm talking about, right? You're watching television, gabbing on the phone, or just puttering around the house—when, suddenly, you're seized with that urge. Visions of microwave popcorn, ice cream, or leftover pizza pop into your head. You try to resist—you remind yourself that you just had dinner two hours ago! Sometimes you're not even really hungry—and yet the call of the kitchen is just too great.

So you give in to that urge. And more often than not, giving in opens the hunger floodgates. "One little snack" leads to another. The next thing you know, you're parked in front of the television set, mindlessly chowing down on all sorts of stuff that's neither good for you nor particularly good.

Fortunately, there's a way to stop this nighttime snacking madness.

The thing of it is, I've been there.

Growing up, I was what they called a "big girl." I wasn't exactly overweight, but I wasn't slender, either. And I wasn't particularly athletic, which meant that whatever I ate tended to show up on my hips, my thighs, my waist.

Nighttime snacks were a major weakness for me. My mother believed in keeping the refrigerator and cupboards stocked to the gills. She also believed in making about six times as much food as we needed for dinner, so we always had leftovers.

In other words, there was never a shortage of snacking material.

Television time was a killer. So was homework time. Many nights after dinner, I'd sit down at the kitchen table to do my algebra or American history homework. And whenever I felt my eyes glaze over or my brain shut down (which was often!), I'd take a break, go to the fridge, and make myself a snack to "keep me going."

Unfortunately, I carried the nighttime snacking habit with me into adulthood. I continued to be a "big girl," and got even bigger. But after I had my son Christopher at age thirty-four, I realized that I was tired of being big. I was tired of not having enough energy, of not being fit. And so I decided to make some changes.

I joined the gym and started exercising religiously. I tried to become more aware of my eating habits— including my way-too-generous serving sizes and my tendency to clean other people's plates—and to re-educate myself about which foods were fattening and which ones were not.

And there was my old nemesis, nighttime snacking. I was still doing it, but with new rationales and excuses. During those evening hours, I allowed myself all sorts of "treats" because I'd had a hard day; because I was feeling stressed out; because I was in a bad or sad or bored mood.

I realized that if I was ever going to lose weight I was going to have to stop eating after dinner. And I did.

My new habits paid off. Over the next year and a half, I lost thirty pounds.

And during that time, one positive change seemed to trigger another. Being able to say no to a late-night bowl of ice cream made me feel good about myself. Feeling good about myself motivated me to exercise more. Exercising more motivated me to stick to a healthy eating plan throughout the day. Sticking to a healthy eating plan throughout the day made it easier to say no to nighttime snacks. And on and on.

In this book, you will learn the tricks and strategies that will help you say no to nighttime snacks. They have worked for me and many others, and I'm confident they'll work for you.

The book is divided into five sections:

- Outsmarting Your Hunger

- Mirror, Mirror

- Finding Your Flow Zone

- Beating the Blues

- Television Time

Each section addresses a different aspect of nighttime snacking, and includes tips on how to ignore and eliminate those bad-for-you cravings.

Also included are three chapters that discuss what to do if you're having a snacking emergency. One offers suggestions for healthy snacking when you absolutely, positively *have* to have *something*. Another chapter provides ways to deal with the social events that keep you out in the evening. And finally, there is a chapter that teaches you how to eat small meals throughout the day so you won't be tempted to eat after dinner.

Read this book cover to cover. Keep it by your side, by the remote, by the refrigerator door. Reach for it whenever you've got the late-night munchies.

Then read it a second time, and a third. There's no such thing as overdoing it when it comes to adopting healthy new habits.

Remember: You're in control of your body. You decide what you eat.

So, take charge and start saying no to nighttime snacks . . . tonight!

Outsmarting Your Hunger

No doubt, you've found yourself at some point having a sandwich and a glass of milk at midnight . . . and wondering, *What am I doing? I'm not hungry, so why am I eating this?*

If you're anything like me, most of the time you're just sort of, kind of, borderline hungry, and you could just as easily go without that late-night snack. Sometimes you're just thirsty and you're misreading the sign for hunger. If that's the case, you should have a tall glass of water or decaffeinated tea. Keep your body hydrated throughout the day so that when you're really hungry you'll know it.

But how do you *not* give in to the siren call of hunger? How do you resist the logic of "Well, I'm just a tiny bit hungry, so what can it hurt to have a tiny snack?"

Remember: It's a slippery slope. A tiny snack can

lead to another tiny snack, until you find yourself chowing down on tiny snacks all night long. And there are many, many snacks that may *look* tiny, but are actually packed with calories and fat. Just take a look at the calorie count of some of the most common evening snacks:

Small bag of Cheez Doodles............190 calories

Four cookies............................200 calories

Slice of frozen pizza....................350 calories

Slice of cheesecake.....................370 calories

Slice of apple pie.......................450 calories

Two scoops of ice cream ....600 calories

So with that in mind, here are 101 helpful tips to keep your hunger at bay till breakfast. I've also included strategies for shopping, meal planning, and rearranging your after-dinner routine so the word *hunger* is totally erased from your evening vocabulary.

1. Just say no!

If you've committed yourself to losing weight, maintaining the weight you've lost, or just plain eating healthier, then make that commitment firm in your mind. If you're reaching for a snack, stop, and tell yourself "No!" Don't have it. Walk away from the refrigerator, sit back down, and pat yourself on the back for your self-discipline.

> *While I was losing weight, my mantra became:*
> *I eat to live; I do not live to eat. This thought*
> *kept me on track and reminded me that I was*
> *in control of my body.*
>
> —Anne, age 32

2. Wait it out for just ten minutes.

If you get the urge to go into the kitchen and "make yourself a little something," wait it out for *just ten minutes*. That's all. Distract yourself by returning phone calls, ironing a shirt for tomorrow, reading a magazine article. Chances are, the urge will pass.

3. Make a deal with yourself.

There's an ice cream bar in the freezer with your name on it. Tell yourself that you can have it tomorrow afternoon. This way, you nip impulse snacking in the bud without feeling deprived.

4. *Brosse-toi les dents,* or brush your teeth!

Do like the French do; floss and brush your teeth right after dinner. There are many reasons why this tactic is so effective: the clean, minty feeling in your mouth will please your taste buds; the thought of going through the rigmarole of brushing and flossing again once you've done it the first time may stop you from eating; and you'll be training your brain with a message: *Teeth brushed, accepting no more food.*

5. Pinch your ears.

Applying pressure to the front of your ears may decrease your appetite, according to reflexologists. The next time you've got the after-dinner munchies, press your finger against the front of your right ear for a few seconds. Do the same with the left.

6. Drink a big, tall glass of ice water.

Not only will it make your stomach feel fuller, but you'll burn calories as your metabolism cranks up in order to heat the chilly H_2O up to body temperature.

According to nutritionists and diet experts alike, you should be drinking eight to ten glasses of water a day. Water is filling, helps flush out toxins, and is great for your skin. Add a slice of lemon or lime for extra zip.

---

7. Pop a mint.

Keep a stash of sugar-free breath mints around. They have almost zero calories, they'll make your breath sweet, and they'll keep your mouth busy so you won't be craving the fattening stuff.

8. Sniff your hunger away.

Research suggests that taking whiffs from a penlike inhaler containing pleasant food scents (such as banana, apple, orange, and peppermint) can help curb your appetite. It's believed that smelling these scents may actually fool your stomach into thinking you're eating real food. Consider buying several—they're affordable and available at health food stores—and keeping them in various snacking hot spots in your house (in the kitchen, on your nightstand, near the television set).

9. Post "no snacking" affirmations.

Get a bunch of Post-Its or a small pad of paper. Write inspiring messages to yourself that you can post on the fridge, *in* the fridge and freezer (especially on snacking land mines like ice cream), in the pantry, and other places where you keep food.

Affirmations can be gentle and nurturing, strong and positive, or tough—whatever works for you:

- "One day at a time"
- "My body is a temple"
- "Just do it"
- "Think before you eat"
- "Is it really worth it?"
- "Do you really want to look like the Goodyear blimp for the rest of your life?"

---

10. Let go of the leftovers.

Cook small portions for dinner, and make sure there are no leftovers. A refrigerator full of leftovers leads to postdinner snacking as surely as day leads to night. It can also lead to the very bad habit of standing at the fridge and scarfing, say, cold spaghetti out of a Tupperware container.

However, if you cook with the intention of making extra for lunch the next day, prepare the leftovers by storing them away so that it's ready to go when you leave for work the next morning. Once they're packaged that way, they suddenly become "off-limits" for the night.

11. Don't buy prepackaged snacks.

This one's based on the same principle as the no-more-leftovers rule: If it's there and ready to eat, you're probably going to eat it. Not to mention the fact that a lot of the prepackaged stuff—even the so-called "healthy" snacks like granola bars, yogurt-covered raisins, and fat-free, sugar-free muffins—are loaded with calories.

> *"I stay away from temptation by not buying anything that's going to tempt me during my weak moments—like while I'm watching Letterman. If I don't buy it, it won't be in the house. And if it's not in the house, I can't eat it."*
>
> —*Jessie, age 27*

12. Talk yourself out of it.

Sometimes, it's just a matter of having a heart-to-heart (or head-to-stomach) dialogue with yourself. The next time you're contemplating an evening snack, ask yourself, "How many calories are we talking here?" "Am I really hungry?" "Can I live without it?"

SCENE: 10:15 P.M. I am standing in front of the refrigerator, having a stare down with a piece of apple pie.

STOMACH: Must . . . have . . . pie.

BRAIN: Yes, but are you really hungry?

STOMACH: Who cares? Must . . . have . . . pie.

BRAIN: Hold on, let's do the math. You'll eat that large piece in five minutes. And a piece of apple pie has about five hundred calories. Is five minutes of pleasure worth five hundred calories? It will take two hours on the treadmill to burn that off.

STOMACH: Huh. Well, when you put it that way . . .

---

13. Make the kitchen off-limits after dinner.

Declare a new policy: The kitchen is closed after dinner. Do the dinner dishes (or better yet, let someone else do them while you unwind with your favorite magazine). Then turn out the kitchen light, shut the door, and keep it shut until morning. Shift the evening's activities away from the kitchen and to other areas of the house: the living room, the bedroom, the bathroom. Visualize your stomach going into hibernation until breakfast.

> *"I do not allow my kids to open the refriger-*
> *ator once we're done with dinner. This is a*
> *habit I want them to learn now while they're*
> *still young. I don't want them to think it's okay*
> *to snack whenever they feel like it."*
> —Leslie, age 46

14. Go to bed earlier.

After dinner, do what you have to do—put the kids to bed, throw a load of clothes in the washer, organize your notes for that early morning meeting—then immediately launch into your bedtime routine. Brush your teeth, wash your face, get into your jammies, curl up with your sweetie or a good book. Lights out by 10:00 P.M. will mean eight-plus hours of sleep, improved mood and energy level, and fewer opportunities for a postdinner chowdown.

15. Remind yourself why you're doing this.

Make a list of your weight-loss and eating-habit goals and post it on the fridge. Seeing your very important goals in black and white every time you reach for a snack will make you think twice.

Possible goals:

- "I want to lose 25 pounds by June."
- "I want to stop eating junk food."
- "I want to start going to the gym three mornings a week."
- "I want to have more energy."
- "I want to fit into my jeans again."

16. Motivate yourself with CDs.

Motivational CDs or tapes such as *Achieving Your Ideal Weight* by Steven Halpern or *Meditations on Weight Loss* by Allen Holmquist may help keep you on track with your weight-loss goals. Such CDs often include tips, inspirational sayings, and relaxing music. Grab one at your local music store or bookstore, or order one online. Then lie down on the couch, close your eyes, and let the motivational good vibes wash over you.

17. Keep a food diary.

It's that all-important A word: Awareness. If you're aware of each and every thing you put into your body, you're more likely to keep the nighttime (as well as daytime) munching in check. Keep a small notebook or food diary with you at all times and record what food you've eaten and how much. Numerous weight management programs make the food journal a mandatory part of their program.

> *"I resisted keeping a food diary for so long because I just found it tedious. But once I started keeping one, and realized how much food I was really eating, I was more aware of what not to eat. It was only then that the weight started coming off."*
>
> —Helen, age 42

Day and time: Monday, 8:40 P.M.

What I ate: Bowl of vanilla fudge ice cream

What I was doing before I ate: Stressing out about work

Before mood: Stressed out!

After mood: Is "fat" a mood?

Fat and calories: 290 calories and 160 grams of fat. Actually, no, because that's for *one* serving, which is like no ice cream at all, so I ate *two* servings. That's 580 calories and 320 grams of fat. Ugh!!!!!!!!!!

18. Reward yourself for not snacking.

Make a deal with yourself that if you can go for a whole week without after-hours munching, you'll treat yourself to a reward. A reward could be a new pair of earrings or a manicure—whatever makes you feel pampered. (Don't use food as a reward, as it undermines your weight-control efforts.) You can adjust the reward system to a reward a day (a long-stemmed rose or half an hour at your favorite Internet site), or a reward a month (a new outfit or a night out on the town).

19. Tell the world!

Announce to everyone—your friends, your significant other, your coworkers, your children—that you've decided to stop eating after dinner because you're committed to improving your health, vitality, and well-being. Share the tips in this book with them. Just talking about it will make you feel more committed to "stick to the program."

20. Do it with a buddy.

It's true what they say—it's always easier to start a new program with someone else. Make a "No Eating After Dinner" pact with a friend and resolve to break old snacking habits together. Check in with each other nightly; set up a joint reward system (movies at the end of the week, shopping spree at the end of the month); and be there for each other when the going gets tough

("Hey, I know it's one A.M., but I'm *this close* to eating a cheese Danish and I need you to talk me out of it!").

21. Kiss someone.

Craving something sweet afterhours? Ask your significant other to eat a piece of chocolate or a bite of ice cream, then enjoy a long, lingering kiss. You'll get the sweet taste without the calories—plus an added bonus!

Mirror, Mirror

L et's face it: We live in a beauty-obsessed culture. Personally, I find this both inspiring and depressing. Seeing gorgeous, hard-bodied women in magazines (or on T.V. or out there in the real world) makes me think that if I stick to my exercise routine, I could look that good! Or, it can make me think: *I'll never look like that, I might as well just stop trying, and, hey, I wonder if that pint of Cherry Garcia is still in the freezer?*

It's a complicated issue. If we were all happy with our appearance—with our body types and sizes—we would be happier in general. We would have more space in our brains to devote to the important stuff, like work, family, relationships, and world peace.

But the truth is, many of us aren't satisfied unless we look good and feel fit. And that isn't necessarily a bad thing. Being attractive and in shape yields genuine, long-lasting benefits that have little to do with looking like a supermodel and a lot to do with health, well-being, confidence, and professional pizzazz.

However images of physical beauty make us feel—good, bad, ugly, or all of the above—we can use them to our advantage. We can use them to make us mindful of where we've been, where we are now, and where we want to go with our *own* physical (and beautiful) selves.

And while we're on the subject of beauty: I've also included some nighttime beautifying rituals for you to try during the evening hours. Because when you pamper your face and body, you look good, you feel good—and, as a result, you're much less likely to spoil all that beauty with a bag of microwave popcorn!

22. Post inspiring images on the fridge.

Are you inspired by images of how you'd *like to look*? Or how you'd like *not to look*? Either way, pick out choice clips from magazines or dig up photos of yourself from your archives. But remember: It's very important to go with what works for *you*. If putting a picture of Cindy Crawford on the fridge is going to send you on a brownie bender from hell, don't do it!

"What finally made me want to lose weight was seeing my vacation pictures. I knew I had

put on some weight, but I didn't realize just how unattractive I looked. So, while I was dieting, I put one of those pictures on the refrigerator. Every time I approached the fridge and saw that photo, it reaffirmed for me the reason to keep dieting—and to not eat after seven P.M."

—Joyce, age 35

23. Watch exercise videos.

The next time you feel like trekking into the kitchen for a little bowl of something, pop an exercise video into the VCR or DVD player instead. You can find them in stores, online, at the library—or, you can tape your favorite exercise shows and keep them on hand for nighttime snacking emergencies.

24. Visualize the end result.

Athletes often use creative visualization techniques before a big event to help them achieve their personal best. For example, a basketball player might visualize herself slam-dunking the ball over and over again, or a runner might visualize himself crossing the finish line first. You can use the same techniques to help you visualize you at *your* personal best.

"To get into the right dieting frame of mind, I bought one of those subliminal tapes. It helped

me visualize myself looking healthy, trim, and sexy. I imagined myself in white shorts and a white midriff T-shirt, looking tan and sleek. This image was imprinted on my brain and every time I considered getting something to munch on, this image would pop into my head and keep my food intake in check."

—*Zoe, age 38*

If you're craving a nighttime snack, close your eyes and . . .

- imagine yourself saying no.

- imagine the numbers on the scale going low, lower, lower still.

- imagine your body slimmer and trimmer.

- imagine doing things you've always dreamed of doing if you could "just shed those extra pounds": signing up for a kayaking class; going to the beach in a bikini; looking fabulous at the high school reunion.

- imagine your friends saying to you, "Wow, you look great!"

25. Plan your future wardrobe.

Tonight, get a pile of clothing catalogs and go window-shopping! Pick out all the wonderful outfits you'll fit into when you lose that weight. Promise to buy yourself at least two.

> *"While I was losing weight, I began collecting magazine pictures of outfits I wanted to wear and looks I wanted to achieve—for when the new me finally emerged. This activity occupied many an evening for me. It crystalized my goals—and the rewards—and kept me on the straight and narrow."*
>
> *—Nicole, age 29*

26. Put mirrors, mirrors everywhere.

Get a bunch of full-length mirrors (available at discount stores for ten to twenty dollars, or keep your eyes open at garage sales). Place them all over the house: in the kitchen, in the bedroom, in the bathroom, in the hallway. Seeing your body at all times will keep you mindful of your weight-loss goals . . . and how to achieve them.

27. Get naked.

When you get the urge to snack, take off all your clothes instead. Take a good, hard look at yourself in the mirror. Remind yourself of how you want to look. Remind yourself of how far you've come. Visualize that muffin you're craving ending up on your hips— forever.

28. Don't cut yourself slack by wearing loose, baggy clothes.

In the evening, change into jeans or an outfit that's very formfitting. It's a lot more difficult to give in to cravings when you're wearing something that hides nothing, has an unforgiving waistline, and leaves "no room to spare."

29. Imagine the love of your life (or the object of your lust) watching you through the window.

Imagine that person watching you as you get up from the couch . . . shuffle over to the fridge . . . grab a slice of cold pizza . . . and scarf it down in ten seconds. Is this how you want that special someone to see you? Would you eat this way in public? Likely not, so why do it at home? Behave and see yourself the way you want others to see you.

30. Create a *Lifestyles of the Rich and Famous* fantasy.

Invest in nice lingerie or a lounging outfit—think silk, satin, or velvet—and make a habit of wearing it in the evening. Sip sparkling water out of a champagne flute. If you look, act, and feel elegant, you'll be less inclined to "spoil the mood" with a late-night raid in the potato chip bag.

31. Do a dry run for a dress-up event.

Is there a special occasion coming up soon—a big date, a holiday bash, a wedding? Spend the evening planning what you'll wear. Try on a bunch of fancy outfits, do your makeup, style your hair. Playing "dress up" and looking glam will distract you from those sneaky snacking urges.

32. Give yourself a steamy, scented bath.

There's nothing like a long, hot soak to make you feel relaxed and beautiful. Pour a few drops of oil under the faucet: your favorite perfumed oil, baby oil, or an aromatherapy oil like eucalyptus, rose, or lavender. Light some candles, play soothing music, and enjoy!

> *"I bought this gorgeous satin and velvet robe that I just nestle into every night. Like the commercial, I said, 'I'm worth it' when I saw the price. And it's that same thought that keeps me from munching away my evenings."*
> —Sophie, age 53

You can have a luxurious herbal bath, courtesy of your spice rack:

- Put two teaspoons each of dried rosemary, mint, and other herbs on a piece of cheesecloth.

- Tie the whole thing up with a string.

- Put the bundle under the tap as you fill the tub.

33. Shape your eyebrows.

The best time to do this is after a bath or shower, when your pores are open. Brush your eyebrows up and then sideways, so you can see their natural shape. Take a pair of tweezers and pluck any straggly hairs along the *bottom* of your eyebrows (not the top) as well as *between* your eyebrows. With a small scissor, trim any long hairs and even out the top. Pluck as little as possible—just enough to give your eyebrows a tamed, together look. Work on one brow first, and then the other, so you can see the difference.

34. Indulge in a home facial.

Put a kettle of water on to boil. In the meantime, wash your face with your favorite cleanser. Rinse. Apply a facial scrub (my personal favorite is apricot) to get rid of dead skin. Rub and rinse. Pour the boiling water from the kettle into a bowl and add a few drops of eucalyptus or other scented oil. A chamomile tea bag works great, too. Then, cover your head with a towel and hold your face over the bowl (not too close!) for five or ten minutes, to let the steam open your pores. Afterward, apply a mask made for your skin type (dry, normal, oily, sensitive), let set, then rinse. Finally, dab astringent on your face with a cotton ball (witch hazel can work in a pinch), then finish the whole thing with a light, soothing moisturizer. You'll feel like a million bucks!

Your refrigerator can be a great source of homemade masks. Try any of the ingredients listed below. Leave on for five to ten minutes and then rinse with cool water.

- crushed cucumber
- mashed, cooked carrot mixed with a little honey
- mashed avocado mixed with a little buttermilk
- crushed fruit (try orange, papaya, pineapple, or banana—or try grated apple with a little honey)
- plain yogurt (or add enough oatmeal to make a paste)
- an egg white

35. Have a manicure.

Okay, enough with the raggedy cuticles and the bare, chipped nails! Have a home manicure basket on hand, complete with cotton balls, nail polish remover, cuticle scissors, cuticle cream, emery boards, and, last but not least, bottles of nail polish in lots of fun, pretty colors: baby pink, sky blue, fire-engine red, lime-green, silver. Get a few bottles with glitter in them, just for the heck of it. Then crank up some tunes or a book on tape and paint away!

> *"This may sound silly, but whenever I felt the urge for some Ben & Jerry's, I would give myself a manicure instead. Since I had to let my nails dry naturally, and I didn't want to spoil the color, I couldn't reach for food. I also had the best nails in my office."*
>
> —Bobbie, age 42

36. Pamper your piggies.

Your feet deserve a break today. Soak them in warm water with a little baby oil thrown in. Massage your feet after drying them off and afterward slough off dead skin with an exfoliating foot peel (available at drugstores and health food stores) or a pumice stone. Next, give yourself a pedicure. Finally, keep your feet oh-so-soft by applying moisturizer on them before going to bed, and then putting on socks. (Feel free to pass on the socks if you've got company!)

To massage your feet:

- Using your thumb, make slow, deep, circular motions up and down each foot.

- Rub the base, middle, and tip of each toe.

- Gently tug on each toe.

- Using the whole hand, knead each foot as if you were kneading bread dough.

- Finish off with light, caressing strokes across both feet.

37. Treat your tresses.

It's not enough to wash your hair every couple of days and get a haircut every six weeks (yes, that's *weeks*—not months!). Spend the evening really lavishing your locks. Give yourself a scalp massage to promote good circulation. Indulge in a deep-conditioning treatment (available at drugstores). And for fun, play around with a different style: go wild with a curling iron; experiment with scrunchies, barrettes, combs, and other accessories; put your hair in a French braid.

38. Brush your body.

Dry-brushing is a terrific way to exfoliate dead skin, stimulate circulation, and make you baby-soft (and super-tingly!) all over. You can buy body brushes at a drugstore or health food store for under ten dollars. Hold the handle and brush firmly but gently all over your body (including back, buttocks, and the backs of your legs). Finish with a light moisturizer.

39. Brush your lips.

Use a toothbrush on dry lips to make them kissable and smooth. Apply a pot of your favorite flavored lip gloss (my personal fave: Kiwi Fruit Lip Balm from The Body Shop).

40. Give yourself a makeover.

If you're in the process of changing your body, why not spend the evening giving yourself a whole new face? If your usual look is understated, go for bold— or vice versa. Experiment by putting blush on your eyelids, dabbing gold powder on your lips, wearing false eyelashes, applying colored mascara (think blue, purple, magenta). While you're at it, throw out yucky old lipsticks and gloppy jars of foundation, and make a shopping list of products you need.

Finding Your
Flow Zone

I don't know about you, but I tend to eat when I'm bored.

Not when I'm *hungry* and bored. Just plain old bored—as in, "Hmm, it's nine P.M., *now* what am I going to do?"—followed by this sort of automatic-pilot trance-induced zombie-march to the kitchen. After which I wander into the living room and polish off my bounty (a bag of nuts, a piece of leftover pizza, an apple). Then I'm on the couch and saying to myself, "Okay, that killed five minutes, *now* what?" Before I know it, the whole ugly cycle repeats itself.

Those evening hours are prime time for boredom to set in. After a nonstop day of work, taking care of the kids, running errands, and making mincemeat of your to-do list, it can be hard to shift into evening mode, which can often be solitary, quiet, and—well, *boring*.

You can beat after-dinner boredom (and the downward snacking spiral that inevitably follows it) by finding your flow zone.

"Flow" is a groovy term that was coined by psychology professor Mihaly Csikszentmihalyi in the 1970s. It has to do with the intense, focused, joyful way you feel when you're performing an activity that you're really, really, *really* into. People can experience flow when they're working, working out, painting, playing the piano, gardening. (A woman I know told me that she's experienced flow while grooming her cat!) The key to flow is finding activities that are challenging but not overwhelming, and then immersing yourself in them with confidence and mindfulness.

Below are a number of activities that may help you find *flow*. Try them, discover your own fun variations, and experiment with new ones of your own. Spend the evening in the zone instead of in the fridge. It's way more satisfying!

41. Exercise!

Exercise will not only help you achieve flow, but it will help you lose weight, feel great, and live longer. Join a gym, find an exercise buddy, invest in exercise tapes, or just put on a pair of jogging shoes and hit the road. Of course, some people find it difficult to fall asleep after an evening workout because their adrenaline levels increase. See what works for you. If you have trouble sleeping after an 8:00 P.M. aerobics class, for example, try a 6:00 P.M. class instead, and eat a light dinner afterward. Remember: If you haven't exercised in a long time, make sure to check in with your doctor before starting a new fitness program. Also, don't exercise immediately after dinner—wait awhile for your digestion to kick in.

Have you thought about trying . . .

- kickboxing
- swimming
- belly dancing
- Pilates
- power yoga
- tennis
- racquetball
- ballroom dancing
- spinning
- weight lifting
- karate
- cross-country skiing
- ballet

---

42. Go for a walk.

Walking is a wonderful way to burn calories, aid digestion, and get you out of the house and away from snacking temptations. After dinner, grab the dog, grab your significant other, grab the kids—or just grab your walking stick and go. Use the opportunity to explore your neighborhood, enjoy nature, or simply get lost in your thoughts.

You can burn approximately one hundred calories by

- running a mile
- hitting the rowing machine for eight minutes
- jumping rope for ten minutes
- riding a bicycle for ten minutes
- playing squash for eleven minutes
- square dancing for sixteen minutes
- playing badminton for twenty minutes
- shooting pool for an hour

---

43. Start that novel you've been thinking about writing.

Tonight, sit down with your laptop (or a legal pad or the back of a napkin) and start your very own great

American novel. Write a paragraph describing the premise. Compose the first line. Compose the last line. Make a list of characters, give them names, and invent backgrounds for them that may have nothing to do with your plot but everything to do with bringing them to life: their childhoods, their first loves, what they do for a living, what they keep in the fridge (hopefully not after-dinner snacks!).

> *"I started writing romance novels when nothing at the bookstore was satisfying me. I would amuse myself by writing a few pages every night until I found myself so caught up in my characters and my story that I was thinking about it all day. Sometimes I would forget to cook at night. Six months later I had a complete novel."*
>
> *—Karen, age 50*

44. Make a to-do list for your house, and then start to-doing.

Make a list of puttering-around-the-house projects that you've been meaning to get to for months (or, in my case, *years*): fixing the sink; cleaning the blinds; putting up the new shower curtain; taking down the storm windows; building a special shelf for the cookbooks. Tackle one project a week and work on it nightly. You'll get *mucho* satisfaction from knowing

that you're improving and beautifying your home—
plus you're not snacking!

Tonight, why don't you go through your closet
and . . .

- bundle up the clothes you haven't worn in years
  to give to the Salvation Army?

- set aside the ones that need mending, dry cleaning, and hand-washing?

- update sweaters and jackets by replacing old
  buttons with groovy, funky antique ones?

- make a list of things you really, desperately
  need—panty hose, a jogging bra, a new skirt for
  work—and then do some online shopping?

---

45. Become an avid reader.

Instead of getting lost in your fridge tonight, get lost
in a book. Pull all the books off your bookshelf that
you've been meaning to read. Or, hit the local bookstore or the library. Ask your friends to recommend
what they're reading. Browse through Amazon.com or
other Internet booksellers. Try something different: a
biography of a famous Hollywood figure; a political
thriller; an Italian novel in translation; a collection of
travel essays.

A great way to become an avid reader is to join a book club—or start your own. If you're hosting, serve a fruit salad. If someone else is hosting, offer to bring one.

46. Learn a new language.

Have you always wanted to *parlez* in French? Order sushi in Japanese? Sign up for a continuing education class or buy foreign-language tapes or videos. For fun, rent foreign movies in the language you're learning. Ignore the subtitles, and see if you can follow along.

47. Do something with your kids.

Evening should be quality time, not snacking time. Tonight, hang out with your kids and do a special activity together. Look at photo albums and reminisce. Make a collage or an "ancestor wall." Draw portraits of each other. Build a LEGO sculpture.

48. Do something with your significant other.

Likewise, spend the evening with your sweetie and really have fun. Make a tape of your favorite songs and give it a silly name ("Music to Procrastinate By"; "Joe and Janie's Top Ten Make-out Tunes"). Play Twister. Play strip poker. Have a conversation that has nothing to do with the kids (or with the bills or with anything vaguely related to real life).

49. Make love, not snacks!

And speaking of having fun with your sweetie . . . spend the evening having sex. Aside from its obvious benefits, it burns a whole lotta calories (we're talking hundreds per hour). Need I say more?

What should you do if the people you live with—your significant other, your kids, your roommate—are die-hard evening snackers?

- Encourage them to follow your excellent example and adopt a "No Eating After Dinner" rule.

- If they still insist on snacking after dark, encourage them to have only healthy stuff like veggies, fruit, or plain, nonfat yogurt.

- Ask them not to pig out in your presence.

- Go into a different room yourself.

- Ask them to keep *their* snacks in distinct, opaque containers.

- And keep *your* hands off of them.

---

50. Dance.

When was the last time you put on some music and just let go? (The last time *I* did that, I was grooving to Donna Summer in my living room, in the dark, in my underwear—and an elderly friend dropped by unexpectedly. But that's another story.) Tonight, slip into something comfortable and crank up the CD player. Put on whatever gets your blood flowing and your feet moving: reggae, hip-hop, jazz, blues. Be the queen of disco. Be the sister of soul. There's nothing like dancing to launch you headfirst (or feetfirst) into the flow zone.

51: Take up astronomy.

Invest in an inexpensive telescope and an amateur astronomy guide and become a true-blue stargazer. Study the sky; learn the names of constellations; become aware of how the stars change position over time.

52. Write letters.

Yes, letters. Buy a box of pretty stationery, or get some engraved with your initials or name and address. Spend the evening writing to three friends you haven't spoken to in years—say, your favorite aunt, your college roommate, and your best friend from high school.

53. Surf the 'Net.

Yes, your boss frowns on it, and it can be a huge distraction if you've got important things to do, but if you have a free evening, it's a great way to pass the time. You can educate yourself about all sorts of subjects; "talk" to people online; and in general become more computer-savvy. Start with a site that interests you. To do a site search by subject, go to a search engine like Yahoo.com or Google.com. Or, go to a general-interest site like Oxygen.com or Salon.com. Then let your whims do the guiding and your fingers do the surfing.

54. Volunteer.

Helping others can stimulate your mind and warm your heart. Think of a cause that's meaningful to you—literacy, domestic-violence prevention, mentoring teens, local politics, the arts—and find out if there's a corresponding institution or nonprofit group in your town. Call and offer your services one night a week. Don't worry if you don't have experience—they will be more than happy to train you in exchange for your time and commitment.

55. Discover your inner artist.

Visit your local art supply store and go crazy: buy finger paints, pastels, tubes of acrylics, cool-looking brushes, pretty tissue paper, colored pencils, enormous drawing pads, glue, glitter. Spend the evening improvising with your fun new supplies. Paint a self-portrait. Do a pastel rendering of the dream you had last night. Glue glitter onto anything and everything. Paint a mural on your bedroom wall.

56. Plan the perfect vacation.

Okay, so you don't exactly have the budget for a villa in Tuscany or a beach house in Bali. Still, it's fun to plan your dream vacation and keep a file for future reference. Do research on the Web; get travel guides out of the library; buy copies of *Travel and Leisure* and *Condé Nast Traveler*; and check out the Sunday travel section of your local paper. It's fun, it's a great way to spend an evening, and, who knows, you may discover that your dream vacation is more affordable than you think.

57. Reinvent your life.

Not entirely happy with your job, with your relationships, with your daily routine? Eager to launch into something new, but not sure how to get started? Spend the evening brainstorming what you *really* want out of life. Don't limit yourself to the predictable or even the possible. Keep a notebook handy and list anything and everything that your heart desires. Then make a plan to achieve the one thing you want most. Staying focused on your goal, whatever it is, is the key to accomplishment.

In his book, *The 15 Second Principle*, author Al Secunda recommends devoting fifteen seconds a day to identifying your dreams, broadening your horizons, and defining new goals. He suggests that people can achieve personal growth by going for "mini-breakthroughs" and "mini-actions" versus big, sweeping, often scary changes. With time, those fifteen seconds per day will multiply to fifteen minutes and then to hours per day as you work toward making your dream a reality.

---

58. Get lost in the library.

I loved doing it as a child, and I love doing it as an adult. Go to the local library—call first to make sure they have evening hours—and just wander around aimlessly, without an agenda. Pick up books at random; check out the audiotape and videotape sections; read magazines and newspapers you've never read before. It's awe inspiring to be surrounded by so many *words*, and it's great to have spontaneous, immediate access to any and all subjects under the sun—for free. Of course, many bookstores these days feel like libraries with seats, couches, tables, play areas for the kids, and even coffee bars. If the library is closed in the evening, the bookstore is the next best thing.

59. Exercise your green thumb.

Gardening is a wonderful way to get into the zone. Peruse gardening catalogs for exotic new plants; or start making plans for next season. If you don't know a perennial from a petunia, pick up a beginner's gardening book and start with a modest, no-brainer garden: for example, a small row of hostas and begonias along the front of your house. If it's the dead of winter, cultivate a windowsill herb garden (think basil, parsley, tarragon, mint) or plant some edible flowers like nasturtiums and violets in pretty hand-painted pots.

60. Sit outside and do . . . nothing.

Okay, so this one kind of goes against the idea of throwing yourself into a stimulating activity. But there's something wonderful and transporting about spending the evening on your porch (or stoop or balcony or front yard) and just hanging out. Listen to night noises; watch people and cars go by; get lost in your thoughts. Be in a different kind of flow zone. Just zone out. And go with the flow.

Beating the Blues

Comfort food. We all know what it is. We've all been there.

The phrase "comfort food" just *sounds* so comforting. And it evokes a world of memories as warm and cozy as a blanket: Mom's meat loaf and mashed potatoes; hot chocolate on a snowy afternoon; cookies and milk late at night, in bed. For me, it's rice. Having spent my childhood in Japan, where rice is a staple, I make a bowl of basmati rice with butter whenever I'm feeling down, depressed, or just plain blah.

There are scientific reasons why so-called "comfort foods" can lift our spirits. Certain foods, especially carbohydrates, actually alter our body's chemistry—including levels of blood sugar and serotonin—and generate quick hits of energy, pleasure, even euphoria.

The problem is, this "comfort" is short-lived. We

feel good for a while, and then we come crashing back down again. We head back to the kitchen for another fix. And all the while, we never address what's really bothering us. Plus, we're not eating out of stomach hunger, but out of head hunger or heart hunger.

Evening is a prime time for bingeing on comfort food. The sun's down, the day's over, and it's easy to feel as dark inside as it is outside. Without busy demands to distract us, we can find ourselves overcome by negative emotions: anxiety ("I'll never finish that assignment on time!"), loneliness ("Everyone's out doing something except me."), low self-esteem ("I'm so fat, I'll never lose that extra weight."). And so we turn to the cookies, English muffins, the leftover macaroni and cheese. Anything to make the inner *dis*comfort go away.

An occasional nosedive into comfort food may be okay. When a friend of mine went through a devastating break up, we went to an ice cream parlor and ordered two enormous hot fudge sundaes for dinner—and nothing else. Under the circumstances, it seemed like the right thing to do.

But in our everyday lives, it's important to distinguish real hunger from our *other* hungers—for a hug, for company, for compassion—and to replace comfort-food strategies with healthier strategies, like the ones below.

61. Determine if you're an emotional eater.

Do you eat when you're stressed out? When you've had a tough day at work? When you're nervous about an upcoming event? When you've had a fight with a loved one? Identifying whether you're an emotional eater is the first step toward curbing nighttime (and daytime) snacking. The next time you've got the post-dinner munchies, ask yourself: "Am I really hungry, or am I just in a bad mood?" If you're just blue, then consider other ways to get out of a funky mood: rent a funny movie, go for a walk, buy some shoes—anything you think will help. And keep in mind that excess, nighttime snacking will only make you feel worse in the long run.

62. Get plenty of sleep.

Studies have shown that sleep deprivation can lead to carbohydrate cravings (not to mention making you tired and cranky, which can lead to other bad-for-you food cravings, too). Make getting a good night's sleep a priority.

If you have trouble getting to sleep, try the following:

- Drink a warm glass of skim milk—tryptophan is a natural sleep-inducer.

- Take a hot bath with lavender salts or oil.

- Put a lavender sachet under your pillow.

- Invest in a better mattress.

- Never work in bed, and don't work right before going to bed.

- Keep the television out of your bedroom.

- Designate the bedroom for sleeping, sex, and reading (books and magazines, not profit-and-loss statements!) only.

63. Call a friend.

Sometimes, what we really need is a sympathetic ear, not a snack. The next time you're feeling blue, fight the impulse to raid the fridge and call someone instead. Chances are, a friendly voice and a good heart-to-heart will take care of what ails you.

64. Deal with the problem head-on.

If you're craving a nighttime comfort snack, first try to determine what's *really* bothering you. Is there something you can do about it (besides numbing out with a bowl of ice cream)? Write down your thoughts ("I hate my job"; "Had a fight with my sister"; "I can't stand the way I look"), and then brainstorm some possible solutions ("Talk to my boss about a promotion"; "Send flowers"; "Call around about gym memberships"). And then do it!

65. Get addicted to a healthy cycle.

Replace the vicious comfort-food cycle (food—short-lived satisfaction—sugar crash—need for more food) with a *healthy* cycle. Get addicted to the cycle of having willpower and resisting bad-for-you foods; losing weight; having people tell you how great you look; and getting a natural high from all that praise and accomplishment.

66. Schedule a weekly night out with your best buds.

Being out with your friends is a surefire cure for the blahs. Go bowling; get your nails done together; go to a concert; go to the drive-in (that way, you won't have to watch the guy next to you scarfing down a bucket of fat-laden popcorn). The possibilities are endless.

> *"For the last ten years, rain or shine, ignoring husbands and children, my two best girlfriends*

> *and I get together for coffee once a week. We go to a local café, have a cup of java, which is constantly being filled, and sit for two hours catching up on the good, bad, and ugly of the week. It's pure therapy. We wipe the slate clean of the week that passed and feel energized to deal with the week ahead."*
>
> *—Virginia, age 34*

67. Host a weekly night in with your best buds.

Another way to guarantee a regular date with your friends is to play host. Play games (think bridge, charades, board games like Monopoly and Clue and Trivial Pursuit); have a discussion group (think *New Yorker* articles; women's issues; weight-loss support); have an old-fashioned quilting bee. Serve a fruit salad and sparkling water.

68. Take a yoga class.

When I took my very first yoga class, I described it to a friend as "exercising and taking a nap at the same time." It's relaxing, it's strengthening, and it always, always lifts my spirits. An added benefit: Whenever I come home from my evening yoga class, my body feels so good and so pure that I don't want to spoil it with a snack!

You can also practice yoga yourself, at home. Get a yoga book or yoga tapes (there's *Baron Baptiste's Power and Precision* or *Ali MacGraw: Yoga Mind and Body*, to name a couple), and an exercise mat or comfortable quilt for floor postures. Add incense, some candles, and some CDs of relaxing, New Age music, and you'll be doing the downward-facing dog and the sun salutation in no time!

69. Give yourself a pep talk.

If you're stressing out about your job or feeling down about your love life, give yourself a pep talk. Sentiments like "It's going to be okay," "I'll get through this," and "It's not as bad as I think" may seem like overused clichés, but they're overused for a reason—because they work!

70. Get lost in the past.

Tonight, curl up on the couch and leaf through diaries, letters, mementos, photographs. It can be uplifting to reconnect with your past self, reminisce about good times, remember old loves and friendships, revel in all the growing up you've done.

71. Get out of the house.

It doesn't matter what for—just get out of the house! Go shopping. Go window-shopping. Go to a movie. Walk around the block.

> *"Whenever I'm bored in the evening and need to get out of the house, I find a reason to go to the local drugstore. I'll go to buy some toothpaste and then spend an hour checking out the latest nail polish colors, eye shadows, hair treatments, whatever. It's fun to look and play with the testers and, strangely, this lifts my spirits. Needless to say, I don't go near the snack isle."*
>
> —*Christine, age 32*

72. Meditate.

Meditation is a terrific and natural way to improve your mood, and it has dozens of other physical and emotional benefits as well. You can do it yourself at home, take a class, or join an informal meditation group in your community.

To practice meditation at home:

- Put on comfortable clothes.

- Find a quiet, private place where you won't be disturbed.

- Sit cross-legged or with your legs in front of you and your back against a wall.

- Close your eyes and breathe very deeply, from your belly. (Your stomach should be going in and out, instead of your chest going up and down.)

- Focus on something repetitive—the in and out of your breath, or a word or phrase you can say over and over in your mind (a "mantra").

- Keep your eyes closed and focus entirely on your breath or your mantra, to the exclusion of everything else.

- If other thoughts enter your mind (and they will!), just imagine the thoughts going into a bubble; mentally watch the bubble floating away; and then return to your breath or mantra.

- Do this for ten minutes or an hour, however long you feel comfortable.

73. Turn to online support.

There are a number of Web sites that provide advice and other types of support (including bulletin boards and live chat rooms) for depression, weight-loss issues, and more. They're available twenty-four hours a day, seven days a week, which can be a godsend if you're feeling comfort cravings at 2:00 A.M. Try iVillage.com, Women.com, and eDiets.com, for starters. Use search engines like Yahoo.com and Google.com to find other sites that might help.

If you suspect that you're suffering from more than everyday blues or short-term stress over a specific problem, you might consider seeking professional help. Ask your family doctor to recommend the names of psychotherapists in your area, or talk to people you know who are in therapy. "Shop around" until you find a therapist or support group you feel comfortable with and negotiate a rate that you can afford. Some insurance plans cover the cost of psychotherapy, at least in part. Check with your insurance provider.

74. Listen to music.

Music really can soothe the soul. Pick out a CD that makes you feel good—Bach's *Goldberg Variations, Al Green's Greatest Hits*, the Beatles, Ella Fitzgerald, Sheryl Crow—and sit back. Really *listen* to the music. Don't do anything else.

75. Inhale.

Beautiful scents have a relaxing, calming effect, and may be just the thing you need for your less-than-ideal mood. Light vanilla, rose, or patchouli candles; burn incense; dab a drop of perfume on your lightbulbs; rub yourself all over with scented lotion.

76. Schedule a massage.

Treating myself to a professional massage always, always makes me feel better, and the good feeling can last for days (and even weeks). If the cost is not in your budget—often forty to eighty dollars per hour, depending on where you live and the type of massage—then consider getting a how-to massage manual and arranging to "trade massages" with a significant other or close friend. You can also massage yourself— use a little unscented oil (or nothing at all) and gently rub your feet, hands, temples, shoulders.

77. Start keeping a journal.

Writing your problems down can help alleviate depression and stress. In fact, "journal therapy" is a growing field, and there are certified journal therapists all across the country. Buy a three-ringed notebook or a bound book with blank pages and start recording your innermost feelings tonight. Remember, this journal is for your eyes only, so feel free to let it all hang out.

78. Practice generosity.

Thinking of others can take you out of your head and away from your troubles. Instead of stewing in your juices (and reaching for the Häagen-Dazs), call an elderly friend and give her the gift of your undivided attention. Go out and buy a present for your mother—just for the heck of it. Write a check (even if it's only for ten dollars) to your favorite charity.

79. Count your blessings.

My yoga teacher told me once that, when I'm feeling blue, I should think about all the things I'm thankful for. My beautiful son. Art. Music. My health. My friends. My fabulous collection of little black dresses. The list goes on and on. And she's right—just acknowledging and being grateful for the *good* things in your life can make the bad stuff seem a little less important.

80. Write a letter—and don't send it.

If someone is the cause of your bad mood—a co-worker, a friend, a family member, your significant other—write that person a letter. Be totally honest, say what you feel, be as angry and nasty as you want. Then rip that letter up or put it away in a safe place.

81. Fill your house with comforting things.

Think big, fluffy pillows. Think cuddly afghan. Think soft, oversized wool sweater. Think bunny slippers. Think beautiful hand-painted tea mugs. Think favorite black-and-white photo (of your special someone, of your child, of yourself as a child) in a pretty frame. Think anything and everything that makes you feel warm, cozy, and happy inside so you won't have to seek comfort in calories.

82. Let it go for tonight.

If you're obsessing about a problem and it's getting you down (and making you hungry), just let it go. Just for tonight. Tomorrow really *is* another day, and you'll have a fresh new perspective in the morning. For tonight, give yourself a break—and save yourself from a comfort-food orgy you'll regret later.

Television Time

There's something about sitting down to watch television that makes us inevitably, automatically think: *Hey, where's the popcorn?*

It's that Pavlovian thing: T.V. time equals snack time. At the first commercial, we're up making ourselves a "little something" to see us through *ER, Ally McBeal, Monday Night Football.*

Haven't you been there? Think about yourself curled up on the couch under the afghan, your eyes glued to the set, your hand making that back-and-forth, back-and-forth trip from the bowl to your mouth. You're dimly, vaguely aware of the taste of popcorn, butter, salt. Mostly, you're just happily numbed out on the double narcotic of T.V. and food.

And of course, even if you manage to *start* your night of T.V. watching without a snack, how can you resist all those yummy food commercials? A sexy couple sharing a pint of ice cream (two spoons, no bowl—so romantic!); a really cute guy polishing off a bag of chips (*he* eats that stuff, and he's got washboard abs!); or a hot, steaming plate of pasta in glorious twenty-three-inch Technicolor (hmm, wonder how long it'll take to microwave that frozen fettuccine Alfredo?). Barraged with these tempting images, how could you *not* make a beeline for the kitchen?

Part of the solution lies in some attitude adjustment. But a large part of the solution lies in learning to do some prime-time multitasking. Many of the following tips will help keep you busy, busy, busy while you watch television so that you won't be distracted by thoughts of food.

83. Don't watch T.V.!

Okay, let's get this one out of the way. Turn off the tube! Your time is precious. So is your body. And we've already established that T.V. watching can lead to serious snacking binges. It's time to replace this spectator sport with something more active and productive.

> *"At one point I realized I was watching at least four hours of T.V. a night. From eight to midnight and sometimes it would run past that because I would be too lazy to get off the*

couch. I thought, what a waste of my time. So I went almost cold turkey. I allowed myself a half hour or one program each night. Suddenly, I was going to bed at eleven, paying my bills on time, finding time to catch up with friends, and even getting in precious exercise time. It was like I woke up after a long hibernation. I should also mention that I found myself five pounds lighter six weeks later."

—Kelly, age 25

84. Put the T.V. far away from the kitchen.

If your kitchen is on the first floor in the back of your house, put the T.V. on the second floor in the *front* of your house. If you live in an itty-bitty apartment where that kind of distance isn't possible, close the kitchen door and put up a DO NOT DISTURB sign. If you live in a *really* itty-bitty apartment and there *is* no separate kitchen, throw a sheet over the fridge instead, and make sure you watch T.V. with your back to the "kitchen area."

85. Get real about food commercials.

Remind yourself that food commercials are exactly that—*commercials*. Eating that pint of ice cream or that bag of chips isn't going to make you happier, make your sex life hotter, or make your problems go away. It's going to make you feel bad and gain weight, and it's going to make the companies that made the food commercials richer. Period.

86. Tape your shows and watch them later.

If your favorite shows have commercials, tape them instead of watching them live. This way, you can fast-forward through the commercials and shave off up to twenty minutes for every hour of programming. You'll not only save yourself from food-ad temptations, but you'll save time, too.

87. Enlist a T.V. buddy and make a no-snack pact.

Invite your significant other, friend, or neighbor to watch T.V. with you. Talk to each other during the commercials instead of getting up to "fix a little something."

> *"I once had a T.V. 'phone buddy.' We'd watch T.V. in our separate apartments, then we'd call each other during the commercials to deconstruct what had just happened. ('Can you* believe *she slept with him?' 'Who do you think killed the husband?' 'I hate that new actress they got to replace what's-her-name.') It was fun, and it kept me too busy to even* think *about snacking."*
>
> *—Nancy, age 39*

88. Catch up on your magazine-reading.

I always keep a pile of magazines on hand while watching T.V. Fashion magazines and other magazines with lots of pictures are perfect for leafing through while keeping one eye on the set. During the commercials, I hit the mute button and breeze through articles, one paragraph at a time.

89. Knock off a few chores.

Is there something in the living room (or den or bedroom or wherever you keep the T.V.) that needs attention? The next time you're watching T.V., knock off a chore at the same time. Dust (*really* dust) your bookshelves. Sand and repaint a windowsill. Pick out new photos for the top of the piano. Take down the curtains and throw them into the wash. Clean out your end table drawers (mine always seem to accumulate mysteriously with pennies, old matchboxes, and Chinese take-out menus).

90. Take up knitting or embroidery or crocheting.

This is a great way to be productive while watching television. Invest in an embroidery kit, a how-to book, some knitting needles or crochet hooks, and several skeins of pretty yarn. (I've often wanted to take up knitting just to buy the yarn—such amazing colors!) Start with a simple project, like baby socks or a scarf.

> *"I credit my knitting with helping me keep my weight down. Not only does this activity keep my hands busy, it also keeps my mind focused on the task at hand instead of what's lurking in the refrigerator."*
>
> —Susan, age 45

91. Clean up your jewelry drawer.

If your jewelry drawer (or box) is anything like mine, it's a tangly, embarrassing, can't-find-anything mess. The next time you're sitting in front of the tube, use the time to untangle necklaces; reunite mismatched earrings; set aside items that need to be cleaned (at home, with warm water and dishwashing detergent and a soft toothbrush, or by a professional, if it's the valuable stuff); pick out outdated pieces to give away or sell; decide if there's a stone or two that could be salvaged and reset as a new ring or necklace.

92. Stretch, stretch, stretch.

Put on a leotard while watching T.V. and do stretching exercises. It feels great, it will get you all relaxed for bedtime, and it nips nasty cravings in the bud.

Some prime prime-time stretches:

- Lie down on the floor, straighten your legs, and stretch your arms over your head. Imagine yourself getting long, long, longer. You can also do this stretch while standing up, like you're a tree growing toward the sky.

- Sit up and extend your legs in front of you. Keep your knees relaxed and slightly bent. Grab your toes, heels, calves—whatever you can reach—and lean forward.

- Sit up and extend your left leg in front of you. Bend your right leg and cross it over your left so the right knee is bent and pointing straight up (while the left leg remains flat along the ground). Grab the outside of your right thigh with your left hand, and pull it toward you, giving it a stretch. Then switch legs.

- Sit upright. Bend your legs so your knees stick out to either side and the soles of your feet are touching. Press down on your knees with your elbows and stretch.

93. Organize your CDs.

Isn't it about time you arranged your impressive CD collection so you can *instantly* find what you're looking for? You could do it alphabetically by artist, by album title, or by category (classical, jazz, blues, rock, etc.). While you're at it, take the time to clean each disk with an inexpensive do-it-yourself cleaning kit.

94. Go for bicep curls, not cheese curls.

There's nothing like exercising with hand weights while you watch T.V. to make you feel virtuous. One-, two-, three-, or five-pound weights work best. If you've never used hand weights before, start with a pair of one-pounders and work your way up. Try bicep curls, tricep kickbacks, chest flies—three sets of twelve each.

For sexier inner thighs:

An ordinary ball (one of those cheap, colorful ones that are the size of basketballs, but softer) can help tone your inner thighs. Lie down on the floor, bend your knees, and "trap" the ball between your thighs (closer to your knees than to your pelvis). Squeeze the ball with your legs very hard, then relax. Do as many as you feel comfortable doing.

---

95. Get out your sewing kit.

Sitting in front of the television is the perfect time to deal (finally!) with holey socks, ripped seams, missing buttons, and fallen hems. Make a pile of clothes-in-distress and work your way through them, program by program.

96. Get out your checkbook.

I hate paying bills. I love watching T.V. So I often combine the two activities. Once a week, I sit down on the couch with a pile of bills, my checkbook, my favorite purple pen (somehow it makes bill-paying less painful), and a wastebasket, and I go to town.

97. Polish your silver.

If you're fortunate enough to have silver cutlery or other nice silver items, take advantage of T.V. time to give them a shine. Buy a bottle of silver cleaner, or try a homemade paste of baking soda and water. Always clean your silver with a soft cloth. Use a soft-bristled toothbrush to get into tough little grooves.

98. Clean out your purse.

This is a great, productive, valuable thing to do while you're channel-surfing. Dump out the contents of your purse onto an old newspaper or a pillowcase. Throw out all the little scraps of what I call "mystery garbage." Throw out pens that no longer work. Throw out those mints that have escaped from their wrappers. Go through your wallet, file important receipts, dump the unimportant ones. Ditto with other people's business cards. Finally, take a soft cloth with a little Windex on it and clean the goop off your makeup containers.

99. Put photos in photo albums.

If you're anything like me, you probably have a huge cardboard box full of photos that you've been meaning to put in albums for the longest time. Why not buy some photo albums, sit down in front of the television, and organize those photos while you watch the latest episode of *Friends*.

100. Crunch, don't munch.

I like to do ab-crunches and ab curls while watching T.V. My personal goal: I'm working my way up to one hundred a day, and eventually, five hundred (à la super model Elle MacPherson).

The perfect ab-crunch:

- Make sure you do crunches while lying on a rug or other soft surface (such as an exercise mat or a thick blanket).

- Lie down with your knees bent and your back flat on the floor.

- Place your hands lightly behind your head, to support your head and neck.

- Keep your eyes focused on the ceiling, on a point that is about six feet in front of you.

- Lift your shoulder blades a few inches off the floor. Breathe out. Do not try to touch your forehead to your knees.

- After a few seconds, lower your shoulder blades back to the floor. Breathe in.

- Do as many as you feel comfortable doing.

---

101. Update your address book or Rolodex.

My address book looks like a two-year-old went through it with a Magic Marker. Not to mention the fact that I don't recognize half the names anymore (old coworkers, old friends, old boyfriends, old almost-boyfriends). Buy a new address book (or Rolodex), sit down in front of the T.V., and transfer relevant names, addresses, phone and fax and pager numbers, E-mail addresses, and other miscellaneous tidbits (like birthdays)—in pencil! Once you're done, toss the outdated info out. Feel a huge sense of accomplishment.

> *"I wanted to put all my business contacts on my new computer program. I didn't have time to do this at work, so I would bring my Rolodex home, log in to my office files, and do one letter a night. Twenty-six nights later, from A to Z, my contacts were input to the computer, and I have twenty-four-hour access to them from home and work."*
>
> —Carmen, age 47

If You Have to Have It

Okay. You've read this entire book cover to cover. You've followed each and every single tip. You've conjured every ounce of willpower you have. But you're still craving an after-dinner snack, and you are absolutely, positively *not* going to bed until you get satisfaction.

In other words: *You just gotta have it!*

First: Try *one last time* to talk yourself out of it. Tell yourself that five minutes of pleasure isn't worth hundreds of calories. Tell yourself that one snack can lead to another, and another, and another. Tell yourself that you've come this far—why blow it now?

But if even that fails, and you still have to have it, here is a list of marginally acceptable, "okay, well, I guess if you *have* to have it" snack suggestions for afterhours:

- fruit (an apple, a banana, a cantaloupe half, a bowl of blueberries or raspberries, a bunch of grapes, a fruit salad made with whatever's in season)

- crudités alone or served with low-cal dip (mix curry powder or dried dill into half a cup of plain nonfat yogurt)

- a fruit smoothie made with orange juice and a banana whipped up in the blender (you can also add frozen berries, nonfat yogurt, skim milk, and/or ice cubes)

- a handful of dried apricots, peaches, or figs

- a dried fruit leather

- a few pretzel rods

- a flavored rice cake

- a couple of dill pickles

- a cup of chicken or veggie bouillon spiked with a lemon wedge and a dash of cayenne pepper

- a cup of tomato soup made with skim milk (or any other low-cal soup)

- a glass of tomato juice mixed with lemon juice, salt and pepper, a dash of Worcestershire sauce, and a dollop of horseradish

- a baked potato topped with salsa (or nonfat plain yogurt and chopped scallions or chives)

- a hard-boiled egg topped with Dijon mustard and a dash of paprika

- a slice of light (low-cal) toast with marmalade

- a half cup of nonfat plain or French vanilla yogurt with sliced fruit and a dollop of honey

- sugar-free instant pudding

- a low-fat frozen fudge bar (just one!)

- a hard candy or lollipop

- hot chocolate

- pumpkin seeds

- air-popped popcorn

Out on the Town

It's one thing to resist the temptations of nighttime snacking when you're at home. *You're* in control of your kitchen, and you can keep a tight rein on what goes in and out of your refrigerator. *You're* in control of your daily routine, and you can make sure your healthy new eating habits are a part of it.

But what happens if you're going out at night? What happens if you're going to a restaurant, to someone's house for dinner, to a party? Faced with the temptations of hors d'oeuvres, bowls of munchies, entrées, and desserts, what's a supposed-former-nighttime-snacking-junkie to do (especially since you'll probably have a bunch of drunk people saying stuff to you, like, "Whassa matter? It's Saturday night! Live a little! Let's order a round of chocolate martinis!")?

Is it possible to stay in control *and* have a good time?

The answer is a resounding yes! In fact, if you pay attention to the following tips, you'll have a better time than everyone else because you'll be keeping your eyes on the prize (that is, a slimmer, trimmer, healthier you) while the rest of the crowd is putting on the pounds.

In general

- Eat a light dinner or a healthy snack *before* you go out, so you'll start the evening feeling full.

- Keep the alcohol consumption to a minimum. Not only will it cloud your judgment ("Let's think, cheesecake must be healthy since it has cheese in it . . . *sure*, I'll have another slice!"), but it has boffo calories: three hundred calories in two and a half ounces of vodka alone (and that's without all the other martini, cosmopolitan, or gimlet ingredients). Better to go with mineral water or diet soda. If you have to drink, order a wine spritzer or a light beer.

- If it's a long evening, alternate alcoholic beverages with nonalcoholic ones (wine spritzer, mineral water, wine spritzer).

At someone's house

- If you've been invited to someone's house for dinner, be a good guest and offer to bring something scrumptious that also happens to be low in calories. That way, you'll know there will be at least one dish you can eat with (moderate) gusto.

- Help yourself to a very small portion of everything. That way, you can have the pleasure of tasting all the courses without overdoing the calories, and you won't offend the host or hostess.

- Eat slowly.

- Do not go for seconds.

At a party

- Stand far away from the buffet and the bar.

- Focus more on the socializing than on the food. Throw yourself into interesting conversations. Get a high off of how good you look and how charming you are.

- Go for the crudités, the fruit, the shrimp cocktail, the smoked salmon. Stay away from dips, chips, sauces, breads, cheeses, sausages, and smoked meats.

- Allow yourself one plate of food—*and that's it.*

At a restaurant

- When you get there, immediately drink a big, tall glass of ice water—it will make you feel full.

- Ask that the bread basket be taken away. If you're with a bunch of bread-lovers, ask them to keep it on their side of the table. If you just can't resist, allow yourself half a roll or a breadstick—but skip the butter or dipping oil, as a compromise.

- Order a glass of wine or a wine spritzer to have with your meal—but no alcohol beforehand.

- Have a green salad (with low-cal dressing on the side or just a little olive oil and vinegar) or a broth-based soup as a first course.

- For your entrée: Go for steamed, roasted, or broiled fish or chicken; pasta with vegetables; grains and beans.

- If you don't see a healthy choice on the menu, ask if you can have something specially prepared: for example, instead of Chicken Piccata (which is chock-full of wine and butter), ask if the chef can make you a piece of broiled chicken without the skin.

- If you *have* to have dessert, see if the restaurant offers fresh fruit or sorbet. If not, how about a decaf cappuccino made with skim milk and a dusting of chocolate on top?

At the movies

- Movie popcorn is an absolute no-no in terms of calories and fat. If your local theater happens to serve air-popped popcorn without butter, that's fine.

- Most theaters have an absurd no-food-from-outside rule, so bringing your own healthy munchies is unfortunately not an option. Some theaters are flexible about this rule if you have health-related dietary restrictions.

- If you absolutely have to buy something at the concession stand, go for the healthiest options possible: mineral water; breath mints; dried fruit; plain pretzels.

How to Eat Throughout the Day so You Won't Eat After Dinner

One of the biggest reasons why people go on binges after dinner is because they haven't fed themselves properly throughout the day. Whenever I have one of those days that begins with sleeping too late, skipping breakfast, running from one meeting to the next existing on coffee and donuts, I get home and it's like, "Oh my God, am I starving or what? Where's that leftover macaroni and cheese?"

We *all* have those days. But even on normal, not-so-crazy days it can still be difficult to eat properly. Who has the time to plan healthy meals, shop, and cook? How can we remember what's bad for us versus what's good for us?

Fortunately, it *is* possible to achieve a well-balanced diet of yummy-tasting foods. Follow these basic guidelines, and you should be able to keep your hunger at bay from sundown to sunup:

Do not skip breakfast. Try some combination of the following:

- a hard- or soft-boiled egg

- wheat toast with a smear of marmalade or jam

- plain, nonfat, or low-fat yogurt with sliced fruit and a sprinkling of low-fat granola

- a big bowl of fresh fruit

- Eat three to five regular meals or six small meals per day. Let your body and metabolism be your guide on this.

- It bears repeating: Drink eight to ten glasses of water per day.

- Keep the caffeine and alcohol intake to a bare minimum. (In addition to all its other negative effects, alcohol has major calories!)

- Try to avoid foods containing added sugar and chemical additives. Whenever possible, aim for fresh ingredients.

- Need I say it? Steer clear of deep-fried foods and fast foods.

For lunch, try some combinaton of the following:

- an omelet made with one egg or two egg whites and loads of sliced mushrooms (use cooking spray instead of butter)

- a bowl of soup (not a cream-based one!)

- a salad of leafy greens, assorted veggies, and low-fat dressing (you can add hard-boiled eggs, chunks of tuna, chicken slices)

- a veggie burger with ketchup, mustard, lettuce, and a slice of tomato on a whole-wheat bun

- a big bowl of fresh fruit

The thing to keep in mind about dinner is that you should have a three-course meal. Have a salad or soup, then have your entrée and finish it off with some fruit for dessert. If you're feeling full at the end of your meal, you're less likely to be hungry two hours later. For dinner, try some combination of the following:

- steamed, broiled, or baked chicken or fish

- black beans, shredded cheese, and salsa wrapped in a flour tortilla

- steamed or stir-fried veggies with brown rice topped with soy sauce, Dijon mustard, and a touch of maple syrup

- a green salad with low-fat dressing

- soup (again, no cream-based ones!)

- mashed potatoes made with skim milk and a touch of fresh garlic

- pasta tossed with steamed veggies and chicken, fresh or dried herbs, and low-fat salad dressing or a tablespoon of extra-virgin olive oil and a little grated cheese

- The trick to delicious, low-fat, low-cal soup is to puree. You can easily sauté chopped red peppers, onions, celery, carrots in one to two tablespoons of oil. Add some cubed potatoes or zucchini for thickness, bring it all to a boil, and, when everything is tender, puree. Use spices for flavor or even some evaporated skim milk if you're really craving the creaminess. A soup like this is not only filling, it's a tonic for your organs.

- There are some schools of thought that say you should go protein-heavy for breakfast and lunch, and carbo-heavy for dinner. Do what works for you. If a protein-protein-carbo combination leaves you craving sweets at night, experiment with a different combination.

- Be realistic about serving sizes. A heaping plate of pasta is *not* a serving size—it's a recipe for serious weight gain. Take your old serving sizes and cut them by a third or by half.

- Eat on salad or dessert-sized plates rather than dinner plates, so your plate looks more full. You'll think you're eating more.

- Eat very s-l-o-w-l-y. Put your fork down between each bite, and chew many, many times.

- Drink a glass of water or have a cup of soup before a meal. You'll feel more full to start with.

- Make the most of your calories. For example, if we're talking one hundred calories, it's better to go with a baked apple filled with raspberries (eight grams of fiber) versus a small slice of angel food cake (zero grams of fiber).

- Become a discriminating (read: picky) eater. If you learn to love fresh ingredients, good cooking, and beautiful presentations, you'll be more likely to feel satisfied after a meal (and not junk out on the junky stuff).

- Never, never eat standing up, on your way out the door, or anywhere but at the table (or at your desk, in a pinch). Always set a place for yourself with a nice plate, a napkin, cutlery, and a glass of ice water.

- When you're eating alone, *just eat*. Don't read, don't open your mail, don't watch T.V., don't even listen to the radio. You'll be more aware of how much you're eating, and how good the food tastes, if you're focusing completely on your meal.

- Get creative with herbs and spices, which have zero calories. You can also zip up blah foods with lemon and lime juice, gourmet vinegars, gourmet mustards, salsas, and fruit chutneys.

- Dare to experiment with ethnic cuisines, which can offer variety without the calories. For example, Japanese buckwheat noodles (soba) can be found in most grocery and health food stores, and are good and good for you. My favorite super-quick soba-salad recipe: Boil noodles for five minutes; drain; rinse in cold water; toss with a tablespoon of gourmet mustard (bourbon molasses mustard works great!); top with whatever sliced veggies you have in the fridge (I like cucumbers and scallions); and serve.

- If you receive a calorie time-bomb gift—chocolate truffles, Christmas cookies, a coffee cake—give it away *immediately*. Take it to a food pantry or to the office (encourage your coworkers to have a feeding frenzy). If worse comes to worst and you have no willing takers, just throw it away—and don't look back.

- And one final bit of wisdom: If you do find yourself totally losing control and going on a major nighttime snacking binge, don't despair! Make up for it the next day by jogging an extra mile or doing extra sit-ups. Reaffirm your commitment to eating well and not snacking after dinner—*starting right now.*

Nancy Butcher writes and edits health-related subjects on the World Wide Web. She is also the author of a number of children's and young adult books.